HE MADE MOVIES BECAUSE THEY WOULDN'T
BELIEVE HIM

A Collection of Medical Stories and Essays

By

BENJAMIN D. GORDON, M.D.

1

ISBN: 978 - 1533661906

FOR MY FATHER

CONTENTS

HE MADE MOVIES BECAUSE THEY WOULDN'T BELIEVE HIM

As a child, my first contact with my father's work was watching home movies of his arthritis patients. A man would be walking with difficulty using a cane; then the same man would be striding easily and confidently. There were men and women. Some started in wheelchairs and then were walking well. He showed these to my mother, my sister and me at our apartment at 555 Ovington Avenue, Brooklyn, N.Y. in 1933. It wasn't until I was in medical school that he could explain to me his theory about rheumatoid arthritis and how and why he treated these patients the way he did. When he told colleagues at medical meetings about his results, no one believed

7

him. Making home movies was a new concept but he realized he needed to learn the skill to validate his claims.

He'd graduated from the University of Maryland Medical School, Class of 1923. (I am Class of 1951.) "Dad', I said, where did you get these ideas about people being sensitized to staph or strep?" In the 1920's, allergy and sensitization were still relatively new concepts. He said he'd read work by a Polish scientist named Besretka (or that's as close as I can come to the name he gave me).

Before antibiotics or steroids, immunotherapy and desensitization were being explored. With allergies, weak doses of a preparation of the allergen, gradually increasing in strength, were found to "desensitize" the patient and relieve the asthma or hives or eczema that was their problem. He learned that people could become sensitized to the proteins of either staphylococcus or streptococcus, the most common infections at that time. From a sinus or throat or tooth infection or abscess, he would obtain a culture in order to make an autologous vaccine. Some people could be extraordinarily sensitive to these proteins. If he found an especially potent strain, he maintained a culture of it in his laboratory at Brooklyn Jewish Hospital to use on a patient from whom he was unable get a culture, enabling an autologous vaccine. I asked how he determined a strain was "potent" and worth keeping.

The culture was grown in broth in the usual way. The broth culture would be put through a filter which would hold back the bacterial bodies; just the exotoxins came through. (Some infectious agents came through the filters, which is why they were referred to as "filterable viruses".) The earliest, a Berkfeld filter, was slow. The later Seitz filter was faster. His criterion for potency of the filtrate was how long an intra-peritoneal injection took to kill a mouse: usually 12 - 24 hours, but a very potent strain would kill in 4 - 6 hours. If unable to get a culture from a patient, he would use a small amount of a potent filtrate as a "detector". 1.0 ml of this filtrate IM would stir up and identify underlying infection. The next day, he'd get a call about a sinus headache or a toothache. If dental exam found an abscess, he would take sterile swabs and a blood agar plate to the dentist's office and culture directly from the infected area. Then he could make an autologous vaccine; the method, at the time, was to use 0.4% formalin on the toxin to make a toxoid. This was in the 1930s and early 1940s. The modern method of toxoid production had not yet been discovered. Attempts to counter staphylococcal infection were made with commercial toxoids such as Lederle's excellent Staph Toxoid #2, my use of which I'll mention later. Antibiotics were not available to the practitioner until late 1945 or early 1946. During WWII, only the Armed Forces had penicillin.

Experience had taught him that some people were extraordinarily sensitive to these proteins in the filtrate. Knowing that the skin is the best antibody-producing organ we have, he did all his work intradermally (ID). This technique (to be described) allowed dosing to be individualized. He emphasized to me the importance of getting the material "into the skin", raising a bleb with the "orange skin" appearance. Injecting subcutaneously was worthless. 0.1 ml ID was the equivalent of 1.0 ml subcutaneously or IM. This way, you could titrate the correct dose for each patient. What he was looking for was erythema 48 hours after the injection. Some people would get this at 0.1 ml ID of a 1:100,000 dilution of staph toxoid. He'd repeat this dose every 2 - 3 days. When erythema decreased, he'd inject

0.2 ml, then 0.3. When there was no erythema at 0.4 ml, he'd go to 1:50,000. If no erythema appeared at 1:100,000, he'd go right to 1:50,000 or 1:25,000 until a response appeared. Thus, he could determine the correct dose for each patient. As the erythematous response appeared regularly, joint swelling began to subside, pain lessened and mobility improved. I've always wondered what alpha or gamma globulin patterns would show with modern electrophoresis as patients were clinically improving. He used the same technique with asthmatics. There was a 7 year old girl who was a severe asthmatic in the Pediatric practice I took over in 1955. Her mother was a nurse and supervised medications needed each night. After six months of using Lederle's Staph Toxoid #2, she couldn't contain her joy at putting her daughter to bed each night without any medication.

One time, when it was my turn to take the Pediatric Service at Bridgeport Hospital, (this was early 1960's) there was a 12 year old girl on the ward with severe Rheumatoid Arthritis. One of the orthopedic surgeons wanted my approval to do a joint stripping, as he did on 50 year olds. When I pointed out she was only 12, he challenged me with "Well, what can you do for her?"

I brought in a vial of Lederle''s Staph toxoid #2 and began ID shots every other day. I had no idea whether she'd respond. After 10 days, she was visibly improved —- and the orthopedist never forgave me. Her pain was gone and her mobility was much better. She was a patient in the hospital's Arthritis Clinic. I called my friends who ran it and asked if they would mind if I continued to treat her in my office. They had not seen her on the Pediatric ward and had no objection. She had gained weight and I sent her back to the clinic after 3 months of toxoid shots. The next day, my friend Dr. Dan Hardenburg called. "What did you do? I've never seen a response like this. She looks wonderful". I told him briefly about my Dad's work.

Dad started the second arthritis clinic in the country at Brooklyn Jewish Hospital in 1932 (the first was at Bellevue in 1931) and opened the Kings County Hospital clinic in 1939. The physicians who worked in his clinics saw these results and patients were beginning to come from all over the country and Canada.

He'd only published one paper in the late 1930's ("The Treatment of Rheumatoid Arthritis With Formalized Streptococcus Filtrate (Toxoid) – Abraham S. Gordon, M.D., Brooklyn, N.Y. – The Journal of Laboratory and Clinical Medicine, vol.22, #6, March 1937) and was collecting the years of cases and experiences when his sudden death from a massive brain hemorrhage occurred in February 1957. Despite all our efforts, he died in 3 days, never having regained consciousness. I read the studies which found the use of IM or subq staph toxoid worthless. They arbitrarily put patients in different dosage groups. These studies were worthless because the appropriate dose for each patient was not determined; i.e., not individualized.

I'd asked him about a major problem: he'd never run a series of controls, using a placebo. He was convinced of the validity of what he was doing by the results he got; it was wrong to deprive patients of relief by giving them plain saline. He said "When all the data were published, the end results would speak of themselves". I was in my second year of solo practice in Pediatrics when he died. His office was in Brooklyn; my practice was in Stratford, CT. I was simply unable to go through the records and data of 20 years of private and clinic work he'd amassed.

One of his most dramatic cases was a little girl named Marcia who'd developed severe rheumatoid arthritis at age 4. Dad first saw her when she was 6. She lived about two blocks from our house on Union Street. He told me, years later, it was not just the toxoid shots but physical therapy, good nutrition and family cooperation that had been important in her recovery. I remember seeing her on the dramatic day, at age 9, holding her older brother's arm, when she walked the two blocks to Dad's office.

Had he lived to collate and publish himself, I think he would have been vindicated.

THE PROPER USE OF HYDROCORTISONE

In 1949, when I was a second-year medical student at the University of Maryland, we were fortunate to have had as a guest lecturer the great Dr. Hans Selye, who had put together the concept of the physiology of reaction to stress or the General Adaptation Syndrome. An Austro-Hungarian who earned doctorates in Medicine and Chemistry in Prague, he attended Johns Hopkins on a Rockefeller Foundation Fellowship and then joined the faculty of McGill. As he knew several languages, and read journals in each one, he became aware that what one group was searching for had been found and published in a different language. Subjecting rats to cold (as the stressor) in his lab at McGill, he saw that the longer the rat was exposed before sacrifice, the smaller the adrenal glands were. They were squeezing out hydrocortisone in their attempt to respond to and compensate for the cold. Death occurred when the adrenals were completely shrunken and unable to provide anymore hormone. He told us that, as clinicians, when presented with a severely ill patient, we must understand and address the concept of stress. *The body may sometimes need more hydrocortisone than its adrenals can supply.* If the patient is to survive, we must help by supplying enough extra hormone to cover the inadequacy. Unless we do this, the antibiotics and intravenous fluids (which were brand new at that time) will not provide rescue. From what I read in today's medical literature, this lesson seems not to have been learned.

I have read of studies providing prednisone for five or six days --- and the conclusion it is not effective. Well, how could it possibly be effective? Prednisone provides the anti-inflammatory effect of the steroid. The "inflammatory response" is our first line of defense. Inhibiting that is the last thing you'd want. The body needs extra hydrocortisone to provide what its own adrenal cortex cannot supply; the hydrocortisone also affects electrolytes (Na, K, Ca) crossing the myocardial membrane. Let me describe a case in point:

I received a call at 7:30 PM on December 26, 1956. This 6 year old girl had been visiting friends and family after the holiday and had come home at 4:00 PM. Her mother said she did not "look good" (a phrase every Pediatrician respects) and took her temperature. 102.4F. She gave her an aspirin and put her to bed. By 7:30, she was in a coma. I told her I'd meet them at the hospital.

She was, indeed, comatose but her neck was rigid. Spinal tap showed leucocytosis and elevated protein. Culture, subsequently, proved Hemophilus influenza meningitis, but that night, flying blind, I had to cover all possibilities with what I had available.

5,000,000 units of aqueous penicillin went into her intravenous fluid and doses of intramuscular streptomycin and chloromycetin were calculated on her body weight. Then I gave her 100 mg of hydrocortisone by slow IV push taking almost ten minutes to inject the dose.

The night lab tech did not like me because I insisted he look up the method for an eosinophile count. Dr. Horace Hodes, from New York's Mt. Sinai Hospital, had recently published a paper showing that a low count would have a favorable prognosis. It was known that hydrocortisone lowered the eosinophiles. If they were down, the body was responding to the stress of the infection. A normal count meant the adrenals had been overwhelmed and prognosis was poor. I left the hospital at 2:00 AM after learning her count was down.

In the morning, she was still comatose and febrile. I gave another IV push of 100 mg of hydrocortisone and, then, attended to other patients, phone calls, house calls and office hours, after which I went back to her bedside. Her parents had been there all day. At 5:30, I gave a third push of hydrocortisone. At 6:30, she opened her eyes, knew her parents, said she was hungry and was afebrile. All three antibiotics were continued for six days., but she got no more

22

hydrocortisone. Obviously, she had been provided with what was physiologically needed according to Selye's dictum.

Knowing that subdural hematoma can sometimes be a late complication of H. flu meningitis, I brought her back to the office a month later for a complete neurological exam. She was fine. Then her mother said to me, "You know, Dr. Gordon, I tried to tell her grandmother how sick she'd been and what a good job you'd done, but my mother said 'if she got so well so quickly, she couldn't have been as sick as the doctor said to begin with'".

My first inclination was to smile with the parents -- since they had been there -- and put it in the category of 'sometimes you just can't win'. But, later, I realized why her grandmother had said that.

In that lady's experience with illness in her lifetime, there were no antibiotics, no intravenous fluids and, certainly, no hydrocortisone. She had only known very serious illness to end in death. If someone survived, they couldn't have been 'that sick'. Some scientist had made the observation that the 20th century had experienced profound changes by the decade as had occurred previously by the century. It was now up to my understanding to bridge a generation gap.

Another experience from Pediatric practice occurred when I was called to stand by during a Cesarean section. I'd watched so many of these I felt I could do one myself. I guess every Pediatrician feels the same way, but that was not to be this time.

This very competent Obstetrician was saying to his assistant "Here's the head --- what is this? This is not the head. It's a fibroid the size of a head. " Pause. "The head and baby are above this. We have to reposition everything."

Towel clips came off the skin. More skin was quickly prepped, towels replaced and the incision lengthened so the baby could be removed. He handed me this limp full-term infant with an Apgar of 4. Vigorous suction of the nose to clear the passages and stimulate respiration, suction of the mouth to clear amniotic fluid and debris and then oxygen. Since the heart rate was slow, I gave adrenaline via the umbilical vein. That stimulated the rate but I was concerned because of the prolonged time in the open uterus and wondered if the fibroid had impaired circulation in any way.

Within five minutes, the heart again began to fade and his color was not good.   This was obviously a situation of stress. Despite being a newborn, I gave 100 mg of IV hydrocortisone again into the umbilical vein. Almost immediately, the heart rate improved -- and maintained. Color better. Sent to the nursery. (There was no Newborn ICU in those days.) Eleven days later, he went home. Physical development was normal but mentally he was "slow".   I was never able to establish whether this was due to his unusual birth experience, genetics or other factors.

The last personal observation of the effect of IV hydrocortisone occurred after I'd left practice and was in full-time ER. What used to be called "electromechanical dissociation" did not occur often. Now called Pulseless Electrical Activity, it is the unusual situation of electrical responses seen on the EKG monitor but no mechanical pulse is felt. Here, also, I used 100 mg of IV hydrocortisone which brought a palpable pulse in 30 seconds. We sent him to ICU instead of to the morgue

ONE FOR THE BOOKS

They did not bring him directly to their home. His adoptive parents brought him from the foundling home to my office with both his ears abscessed and running pus. He was six months old.

We did not have the range of antibiotics available today. There were only seven besides the sulfa drugs: penicillin, streptomycin, erythromycin, oxytetracycline, chlortetracycline, tetracycline and chloramphenicol. Knowing how they interacted was crucial: some combinations were potentiating but some, we'd learned to our dismay, were antagonistic. I cleaned out his ears and nose and prescribed a combination that usually worked well on severe ear infections. He cleared nicely. I was especially pleased at the good response because they had had such extraordinary medical problems with their first adopted child. She'd had severe recurrent kidney infection.

Because of the anatomical structuring of the eustachian tube in children, they develop ear infections more easily than adults. So it was not surprising that he had more ear infections during the next two years. I went over the causes of repeated ear infections at this age: possible underlying allergies, an excess of dust - and possibly a dust allergy, parental smoking which irritates tender mucous membranes, sibling or parental chronic infection (more than once had I sent a parent to have infected tonsils removed because they were feeding infection to the child though they themselves might not be acutely sick), or acquired immunologic deficiencies such as acquired hypogammaglobulinemia.

At 2 1/2, after six ear infections in six months, we removed his adenoids. Two months later, he had an ear infection. I used antibiotics based on cultures of his ear pus. My ENT colleague had taught me how to properly lance an eardrum to relieve the pressure and pain and to evacuate the pus. I had become an expert - though not on this boy alone. It is a common Pediatric problem. It was gratifying to see a baby asleep on its mother's shoulder after a myringotomy when it had been screaming in pain on arrival.

At 3 1/2, because of continued recurrences, we removed his tonsils. Since tonsils and adenoids are lymphoid tissue, which helps the body build immunity, we did not remove both the first time to leave him as much immunity-building capacity as possible. The indications for their removal are (1) when the tissues become so loaded with infection that they no longer protect but are spilling infection into the system and (2) when they are so large they obstruct breathing passages.

Two months later, he had another ear infection. I searched the textbooks for esoteric causes. I sent him to local and university consultants. Then, one September afternoon, when he was five years old, I got the call I'd been dreading:

"Doctor, you'd better come right over. He just got up from a nap and he's sitting at the table just staring to one side and he won't answer me." I said, "You get him to the hospital immediately. I'll meet you there." I was correct in my anticipation of a long and desperate night.

Yes. His ears were infected and full of pus. By this time, he was in a coma. What was well-known in the days before antibiotics was that repeated ear abscesses could erode the bone of the roof of the middle ear cavity and spill into the brain. Either this or spill into the mastoid cells behind the ear. Though this was not seen much anymore, I remembered stories of my younger sister who almost died this way back in the early thirties. My father was a doctor, my mother a nurse. When I was in medical school, they described what they had been through with her before she was a year old: ear abscesses, pneumonia, oxygen tents. Opening the eardrum to evacuate the pus was all that could be done at that time. There were no antibiotics. Both of them had seen babies die. Their professional colleagues knew better than to try platitudes. It didn't take much to

30

imagine the nightmare of agony and worry they had been through until her mastoid surgery at age two. Now I was looking at the same potential situation in my patient and could empathize with these parents better than they knew.

I called a neurosurgeon in consultation. On the phone I said "Stan, I don't want to do a spinal tap because he obviously has increased intracranial pressure and his brain may herniate. Can you see if he has a brain abscess you can evacuate?" He came in immediately.

In the meantime, I had blood tests and cultures done and was giving him antibiotics intravenously and intramuscularly. Then he stopped breathing. He was in a private room at the back of the old ward. Facilities were not what they are now. I saw his father's anxious, pale face at the door. I told him to get the nurse while I started chest resuscitation. She put oxygen over his face as I continued to work on his chest. In retrospect, the things that flash through one's mind at critical times are

31

always a source of amazement. Two thoughts came to me as I was fighting for his life: the first was that this boy, his father and I all shared the same first name; the second was my father's words when we talked about antibiotics. He'd said "You're going to be able to save people I had to watch die." Dad, I thought, I hope you're right this time. The neurosurgeon arrived just as the child began to breathe on his own again.

We took him to the operating room for a diagnostic study to see if we could locate an abscess. By now, it was after 9:00PM. When we had the x-rays, my friend delivered the coup de grace: "I'm afraid I can't be your hero tonight. The pressure on the right side of the brain is not localized. There's no abscess to drain. It's a cerebritis- a cellulitis of the brain. The entire hemisphere is inflamed. Your antibiotic therapy is going to have to save him. I'm sorry. I can't do anything more." And he left.

I had researched the subject of antibiotic synergism and antagonism during my senior year of residency and now drew on every bit of information I'd uncovered. I increased the intravenous dose of penicillin and pushed the others as high as I dared. I talked with the parents who, over the years, had become friends. This night we formed a special bond. It was 2:00AM before I thought his breathing looked stable and I felt it safe to leave.

When I arrived at the ward the next morning, he was awake and taking sips of fluid. On the third day, he was riding a tricycle around the ward. I thought "If there was a hidden pocket of infection anywhere causing his recurrent infections, it has to have been eradicated with the intensive therapy he'd received. He went home after a week.

One month later, he was in my office with an ear infection. I sent him to the university consultant again with a detailed account of the hospital episode. The consultation produced only sympathy at my frustration to find a cause for the recurrent infections.

Two months later, I saw he was again scheduled for an office visit. While I was writing up the record on the patient just before him, the examining door flew open and my nurse came in wildly excited. "I just found out why he's having all those ear infections." She was an excellent clinical nurse with twenty-five years of experience. We had been through these past years of frustration together. I did not take her pronouncement lightly.

"Okay", I said. "Hit me with it. What's the explanation I've been missing? What is it I haven't thought of?" Her answer was one more supporting strut for the old adage "A little knowledge is a dangerous thing".

Years before, I had explained to his mother that dust allergy could irritate mucous membranes, upsetting their normal resistant status and increasing susceptibility to infection.

Whenever I told this to mothers, they would usually vacuum extra thoroughly to reduce dust to a minimum. This woman, who was very bright and dynamic, had heard that doctors treated allergy by repeatedly exposing a person to small amounts of the same substance. What she did not know was that this was done by preparing a specific vaccine for each individual and was given by injection. Doses were determined by a trained allergist. She, however, had decided to do this on her own. In the waiting-room, making woman to woman talk with my nurse, she was complaining about how hard she worked and had said "--- and by the time I finish vacuuming the house and dumping the dust in his room ---".

My nurse came out of her chair with her mouth open and her eyes wide.

"You do WHAT?"

"Oh, yes", she said. Years before, when I had discussed the possible role of dust allergy, she had decided to dump the dust in the child's room every day to repeatedly expose him to it in case it might be a factor. It had become such a part of her routine, she did it automatically. When I now realized to what this child had been subjected, I marveled at his being free of infection for 1 -2 months at a time.

I persuaded her to stop this immediately and referred her to a competent allergist. The recurrences came to an abrupt end.

In medicine, we use differential diagnostic exercises for learning and stimulation. I have often thought that this etiology was really "one for the books".

OF ALL THINGS ----

She was 12 years old. Her mother called me because
she'd had fever for the last five days; not continually,
though. It had been normal on the third day but
returned these last two days. This was the summer of
1959. I admitted her to the hospital since it was the
classical picture of a septicemia. My task was to find
the cause and cure it.

Complete physical exam on admission revealed only
some redness in the tonsillar areas and nothing else.
Blood count, urinanalysis, blood culture and all the
esoteric tests were negative. She had no rash. Despite
her flexible neck, I did a spinal tap. Exam and culture
there were also negative. The only odd lab finding was
a normal sedimentation rate, which should have been
elevated. The professors in medical school always said
"Make a diagnosis based on what you have". My father
had taught "when you have a problem, go back to
basics".

So what did I have: a child with a septic fever, some tonsillar inflammation and an inappropriate lab finding.

I decided to go to the hospital's library and look for a text of bacteriology written before antibiotics were available. I found one published in 1945 and went to the section on Septicemia. Perhaps the natural history written by someone who was unable to interfere with its course, using the new medications, would give me a clue.

The text on Septicemia had all the things I'd expected. Nothing unusual. I was about to close the book when my eye caught a small paragraph labeled "Addendum". This said that, rarely, septicemia could be caused by a staph albus, usually thought to be a non-pathogen. A phlebitis in the tonsillar area allowed access to the blood stream and it would then lodge in the bone marrow.

In those days, we did everything ourselves. I'd done a Rotating Internship and one year of residency at Kings County Hospital in Brooklyn. About the only thing we didn't do at the bedside was drain a subdural

38

hematoma. The surgical supply room sent down a bone marrow aspiration kit but, before performing this, I went to the Bacteriology lab and got a blood agar plate and sterile swabs. I inoculated the first aspirate of marrow directly onto blood agar and streaked it out. After my residency, and before starting private practice, I'd spent a year doing research in the immunology of streptococcal disease and Rheumatic Fever so I was familiar with inoculating blood agar plates. After the culture, I made the usual marrow slides. I did not start any treatment since I had no diagnosis. "Blind treatment" might only confuse the picture.

Next day, the lab called. "We're sorry, Dr. Gordon. We don't have an answer for you. The marrow culture only grew a staph albus." My elation at the diagnosis, however, was short-lived. How do I treat something I can't look up or on which there is no one to consult.

I remembered something valuable I'd learned from a friend's casual remark about a patient I had one morning during my internship when I was on the ENT service. The patient was 35 years old and had a marked cellulitis of the neck. In those days, we only had a limited number of antibiotics besides the sulfa drugs: penicillin, streptomycin, terramycin, aureomycin, declomycin and chloromycetin. I was understandably worried about him when one of my passing friends mentioned that aqueous penicillin could be given intravenously in huge doses such as 3 - 5 million units in 500 cc of D/W or D/S. I decided to be 'heroic' in view of this patient's history. I didn't know anything special from the initial routine history but when I did a venapuncture to draw admission blood tests, he passed out. Well, I thought, some people react that way to needles; but when he awoke, he apologized to me. I began to reassure him no apology was needed but he interrupted me.

"No. You don't understand. My concentration camp was one of those where human experiments were done. As prisoners, we were, literally, lab animals. A doctor, coming across the camp, might take it into his head to wonder what would happen if he scooped up some dirt, put it in some fluid and injected it into someone's vein. When one of them came at us with a needle, we never knew if we might be dead the next minute. I knew you weren't going to hurt me but the memory of what could happen with a needle in my arm -----."

I was horrified. Before I could say anything, he asked if I'd noticed the round scars on his back. He told me "Those are from the dog's teeth". I just looked at him. It seems one of the 'amusements' of the Nazi officers was to starve several big dogs for a day, have some prisoners strip to the waist, send them running in the woods and then release the hungry dogs to go after them. Somehow, he had survived this, too. More than ever, I did not want him to succumb to cellulitis in the Land of the Free.

Intravenous aqueous penicillin worked beautifully. Neck swelling and fever were gone the next day

Later, I used this on other cases with excellent results. That's why I decided to try it on this septicemic young girl. 5,000,000 units were put in 1000 cc of D/S and set to a rate that would last 8 hours.

41

The next day, there was no fever but, of course, I ordered the same on the second day. Again, there was no fever. Now the decision had to be "for how long do I do this?' There were no guidelines. The decision to stop was made after six afebrile days. She was feeling fine and was discharged on the seventh day. The fever never recurred --- and my payment never materialized. Her parents absolutely refused to pay me.

At first, I was amazed and unable to understand. Later, I thought of a possible explanation but --- one can never be sure. They never brought her to the office afterwards and I never saw her again.

Oh, yes! I still remember her name.

IT'S BASIC TO DRAIN AN ABSCESS

In the early days, when I started practicing Pediatrics, using an ear curette was essential to be able to see the eardrum. I quickly found how frequently the most common pediatric infection, otitis media, was purulent. These were properly referred to a competent ENT surgeon for myringotomy.

After two years, his practice was getting busier and the babies, being urgent, were playing havoc with his office schedule. "Why don't I teach you to do these as I teach my residents. You'll need an operative head on your otoscope, a myringotomy knife and a knowledge of middle ear anatomy. Bisect the eardrum horizontally and always stay below the "equator". The handle of the malleus you see is the lowest point. All the ossicles are above this."

The first time I did one, I found that a gentle jiggling of the knife would slit the tympanic membrane easily. What amazed me was the speed and force with which the pus rushed up the canal; and the obvious change in the child's crying with release of the pressure.

43

Another ENT, discussing his technique, taught me to suction the pus and clean out the middle ear. The suction machines I had in each exam room were mainly to clear nasal passages. Embryologically, the nose is part of the respiratory system and the mouth part of the GI system. Though we learn to mouth-breathe with a stuffy nose, an infant still functions instinctively, always struggling to breathe through the nose. I always taught parents to use a 3 oz size ear syringe for nasal suction, slightly lifting the tip of the nose to suction along the floor, which is the intake passage. (Note: years ago, a clever ENT did a 'nice' experiment, since it made the point so clearly. Despite the fact that the nasal passage is one cavity, he noticed, with his own breathing, that intake was along the floor of the nose but, to feel exhalation, he had to place his hand in front of his upper lip. Realizing that exhaled air was a weak acid -- $CO_2+H_2O=H_2CO_3$ -- he placed litmus paper cut to the shape of the entire septum. The area along the bottom, opposite the inferior concha, remained pink but the portion on the upper part turned blue. Exhaled air hit's the roof of the nasopharynx and then is forced down and out.) My friend's advice for effective

44

removal of middle ear contents was to cut off the last six inches of the suction catheter, removing the side holes, leaving only one hole at the end. This worked very well. However, I never ceased to be amazed at how much pus came out of those little ears. I must admit, though, that my heart was in my mouth for the first few hundred myringotomies before confidence reigned. To be a good doctor, you have to gird your gut and do what will be best for your patient. Anyone who can't manage this is in the wrong field. With the nasal passages cleared and the pressure gone from the ears, the child was usually asleep on its mother's shoulder before the prescription was written.

Every ear was checked a week later. The clean slit of the incision allowed good repair. No one ever had hearing problems except for the unusual case described elsewhere ("ONE FOR THE BOOKS"). Most pus was typical but, occasionally, as I withdrew the suction catheter, I'd find pus that was very thick and reminded me of the mucilage we used as children from those bottles with the slanted rubber tops. This was, obviously, what the old clinicians referred to as a "glue ear". Unfortunately, I never had culture material available to determine the organism causing this.

A point of technique: in doing an I & D anywhere else -- an arm or on the back -- the proper method is to insert a probe and rotate it throughout the cavity to break down the septa that form, creating a single cavity with no pockets of pus left anywhere. This can be flushed with peroxide or saline and packed with gauze to allow healing from the bottom up. Since this is impossible with a middle ear, you must be alert to the tendency of an abscess to form septa. On occasion, after the myringotomy and suction, re-examination would reveal another area of pus which required a second or third incision and suction. This is one of the "devilish details" but, if attended to, will give the reward of excellent healing.

ADENOIDAL ABSCESSES

In one of the very early issues of Pediatric Clinics of North America, I saw an article entitled "Chronic Suppurative Adenoiditis". Knowing that this publication selected only top quality material, I read it carefully. It proved to be one of the most valuable monographs I'd ever read and gave me the means to cure many instances of a most frustrating problem: chronic night cough.

An irritating night cough grates on the whole family. ENT exams and x-rays (in the days before CT scans) would be negative. Since pulmonary pathology will cause cough day and night, this had to have another origin. The actual syndrome was described by no less a physician than the great Dr. Emmanuel Libman. The story told in the article was this:

Libman had a man with this complaint in the 1930's. He did every diagnostic procedure available at the time. All were negative. Then, in what was described as a typical maneuver for him, he made himself sit down with an anatomy chart and put his finger on each part to see if there was any area about which he had no information: he hadn't inspected, palpated, percussed, auscultated or x-rayed. The only place was the nasopharynx.

Putting on a glove, he reached up behind the uvula and palpated abscesses in both adenoidal areas, which he proceeded to press and break. An enormous amount of mucopurulent material was coughed up and blown out. He made smears from his glove and demonstrated polys and cocci. There was no doubt these were abscesses. (I did the same thing the first time and confirm this finding.) As I began to look for this in cases of chronic night cough, I discovered another diagnostic sign of this syndrome: a frankly purulent discharge on the floor of each nostril.

The first time I decided to digitally explore the nasopharynx of a child, I was guided by one of the basic tenets of Pediatrics: prevention. I put together a pile of tongue depressors and made sure it was slightly thicker than my finger. Telling the child to "Open wide", I put this between his molars before putting my finger in his mouth. Having him take four deep breaths first, I quickly put my finger up behind the uvula and, sure enough, there were the abscess masses. It only took a few seconds to press firmly into each one and break it. My nurse was ready with a basin to catch the large amount of purulent mucus. One of the most dramatic episodes was with a 10 year old boy. After he had finished ridding himself of the abscess contents, he picked his head up, opened his eyes wide and blurted out: "Wow! I can breathe."

Over the years, it was "seek and ye shall find". Eventually, I was able to provide parents with information about what to expect. Being able to anticipate a course of recovery for a patient can make things much easier for them. Occasionally, it was as though a magic wand had been waved and the cough was gone that night. More often, there was gradual reduction before disappearance which could take between 3 - 7 days. Ancillary instructions included steam inhalations to keep the residual material soft so it could be eliminated. The heat would also keep blood vessels open and inhibit bacterial growth. Cough preparations were only those with ingredients to keep the mucus thin (expectorants). "Drying" preparations and suppressants were to be avoided.

These patients are not sick enough to be hospitalized but months of night cough can stress any family.

Nowadays, with scopes that can directly examine the nasopharynx, these can probably be diagnosed and eliminated under direct vision with constant suction. However, any doctor who might find themselves in a situation without modern ENT equipment should remember they're not helpless.

BELLYACHE

A child's complaint of abdominal pain is always worrisome because it is, so often, insignificant. But what if ----.   Exactly because it is a child, you don't want to miss ---;   and especially if it's a friend's child. This was 1962. No CT scans or ultrasound.   Clinical skills.

These good friends called one afternoon because their 10 year old son was complaining of abdominal pain: steady pain, periumbilical, no nausea or vomiting, no diarrhea, no dysuria, no fever, no respiratory symptoms or cough. (A vision of an Attending Physician shaking his finger at the class: "Don't forget that right middle lobe pneumonia can cause right-sided abdominal pain." Not something you'd want to miss in a friend's child.)

"Meet me at the ER."

His color was normal. He walked and climbed onto the exam table with ease, but his face was anxious and worried. There was no question: he hurt.

Ears, nose, throat, breath sounds, heart –
normal.

Abdomen   tender everywhere but no guarding,
no rebound, no history of starting centrally and moving
to the right lower quadrant. Sensation and reflexes
normal -- as I remembered a grinning neurosurgical
resident saying "You Pedes always forget that a dorsal
nerve root tumor can cause abdominal pain."
Something else you would not want to miss in a friend's
child. Keep Zoster in the back of your mind before the
rash appears. No sign of trauma.

The blood count was normal: no anemia or
elevated white cell count. Urine clear. Rarities like
abdominal epilepsy flicker through my consciousness,
which I have found several times. We'd need to do
stool cultures and studies for parasites. There was no
sign of or history of a spider bite --- but, then, that
causes a rigid abdomen, which he did not have.

I was hoping he would not be the third, after
two famous cases I'd had with a surgical friend. This
doctor was not only "the boy with the golden hands"

but had equal clinical diagnostic skills. The first of those cases had what I thought was acute appendicitis, and he'd agreed; but, as we waited for the blood test confirmation, all signs disappeared and the blood count was normal. By the tenth episode, we agreed on a course of action remembering the surgical dictum of the previous generation: "You don't know and I don't know. Give me a knife and I'll find out."   And that was exactly what had happened. The child had a congenital fibrous band that went from the tip of the appendix to the caecum. Peristaltic waves occasionally twisted and strangulated the appendix causing the classical signs and symptoms. The further peristalsis unwound it and all was gone. After the appendix and band were removed, he never had another episode. On the second case, he operated after six ER trips – with the same finding. But, somehow, I didn't feel this child would be the third case.

As we all know, with time and experience, your unconscious will tickle your intellect and you should just go with it.

As I stood there reviewing possibilities, something distracted me from the academic. Turning to this young man, whom I knew well, I said " Jared! What did you eat?"

Eyes looking down at his feet, shoulders shifting uncomfortably, looking at me, then at his folks ---- and then the story came out.

He loved coffee cake. When no one was around, he went to the freezer and found a coffee cake --- and ate the entire thing, still SOLIDLY FROZEN.

And whaddya know! He had a bellyache.

HAIR LOSS TRACED BACK TO BATAAN

One evening I'd signed out to a friend I knew to be a competent Pediatrician. The next morning, I found that one of my patients, a 12 year old girl, was in the hospital after having had surgery for a ruptured appendix. This surprised me, although we all know that diagnosing appendicitis in a child can be tricky. This was 1959. Only a few antibiotics were available. She remained in the hospital four weeks.

Two weeks into her stay, one of the nurses took me aside and provided previously unknown information. She was a relative and had been at the house that night. Though she was a nurse, she was unable to interfere as she heard the father playing down the child's complaints; she wanted me to know that the other doctor had not been given accurate information. This was why care had been delayed until the appendix had ruptured. I was glad to know this was not my colleague's fault but tucked the father's behavior into a corner of my memory.

She was sent home in good condition after the four weeks.

One month later, her mother called to ask why this healthy 12 year old was losing her hair. Before she arrived for her appointment, I did my homework with a text of Pediatric differential diagnosis. What could possibly cause this? She was not hypothyroid. She'd had no contact with a thallium rodenticide. Hypervitaminosis A?

Taking a history during her visit, the following information was revealed:

Her father had been with the American troops on Bataan peninsula in April 1942 when they'd had to surrender to the Japanese Army. They could not be supplied or reinforced; they were weak, malnourished and diseased, and there were so many more prisoners – Filipinos and Americans – than the Japs had expected. The Japanese commander, General Homma, knew that the U.S. troops defending the city of Corregidor expected a siege (i.e., blockade and bombardment) but he was planning an amphibious attack. Not wanting to let the prisoners see him training troops for this tactic, in case some escaped, he decided they had to be moved. Since vehicles and gasoline were not available in sufficient quantity, he ordered them to be marched 80 miles to Camp O'Donnell. That march is one of the grossest horrors in human history. The prisoners were beaten, tortured, beheaded and starved. Japanese culture taught that it was dishonorable to be defeated so they considered their charges "less than human".   In addition, there were 78,000 prisoners when the Japs had expected only 25,000. Anyone lagging behind was bayonetted or shot, beaten or tortured.   My patient's father was one of the few surviving Americans to reach Camp O'Donnell and, somehow, survive until the end of the war. As you can imagine, all survivors were "nuts" about good nutrition.

Her post-operative course was not an easy one. She developed an abdominal abscess, which was not an unusual complication after a ruptured Ap in those days. With memories of his experience 17 years before, he was going to be sure his child had proper nutrition.

When the mother showed me what her daughter was taking, the diagnosis became clear. The recommended dose of vitamin A for a girl her age was 800 micrograms daily. She was a good eater and liked yellow and green leafy vegetables --- but was getting 50,000 micrograms daily, as well as overdoses of everything else.

It took patient explanation to get the father to understand that both vitamins A and D were among the fat-soluble vitamins and were stored in the body. Excess amounts did not just wash out as did vitamin C and the B vitamins, though even some of the latter could be problematic. He was unaware that there were known syndromes of overdosage of both A and D, hair loss from A being well-known.

He was reluctant to take my suggestion to stop all vitamins for, at least, three weeks, but eventually did agree – and was more comfortable with the decision when her hair loss stopped and she was just fine.

THE TREATMENT OF BURNS

They brought him to the office (before the days of full-time ER staffs) with a large severe second-degree burn of most of his lower abdomen. His grandfather had made him a cup of tea and placed it on the table. Being three years old, and knowing it was for him, he reached for it --- and spilled it on himself.

I cleaned it with zephiran (which we used before there was betadine) and covered it with Furacin ointment before putting on Vaseline gauze and a dry dressing. I don't know when I started using what I came to call a "window dressing"; i.e., taping the four sides of the bandage to the skin so no dirt could get to the wound but leaving the center of the gauze exposed for aeration.

At his return in three days, I started the usual method at the time: removing the dressing to place a new one. His crying from pain as I began made me re-think. The real goal is to prevent infection: so I left the Vaseline gauze in place, cleaned over it with zephiran and peroxide (to inhibit anaerobes), placed more Furacin and re-dressed it.

On his next visit, several days later, the area looked clean and, without too much thought about it, I cut away gauze on the periphery which had loosened. Repeated infection control technique as before. Then, at each visit, I was aware that I was cutting away gauze at the periphery and the skin, as I uncovered it, was perfectly normal. As the size of the burn area reduced, it was gratifying to see normal skin, only now I was becoming aware that this had been part of the original burned area. It was healing *without scar formation.*
At the last visit, when the top gauze dressing was removed, there was nothing to cut away. The last bit of Vaseline gauze was just sitting on the skin --- skin which was completely normal.

All burns and deep abrasions thereafter, were treated the same way -- with the same results. At one point, I tried to tell this experience to surgical friends --- only to be met with polite condescension. The unspoken message was clear: "You're not a surgeon. How could you possibly know something of value to us?" But it works. As the old commercial used to say: "Try it. You'll like it."

TWO REMEMBERS
GENE A.

He was a five year old on the Pediatric Service
when I was a rotating intern at Kings County
Hospital in Brooklyn, N.Y. in 1951. He had
leukemia and had been transferred to KCH from
Greenpoint Hospital, though, at that time, there
wasn't much more we could do. He was bright,
perky and handsome. A real alpha. My wife would
join me after her work to visit and play with him.
Anything he didn't like was "stinky poo". There
was no family. His mother would visit but she had
had him out of wedlock before she'd met her
husband and was terrified this might be discovered.

I went to Greenpoint Hospital to summarize his
records there. Did they remember him?

Oh, yes! One suppertime, he didn't want to drink
his milk. Looking around, he decided a certain box
near the floor would be a good place to dispose of
it. He dumped his milk in what turned out to be a
main fuse box and short-circuited half the hospital.
"Oh, yes! We remember Gene." He died two
months later.

POLITICAL SECRET

It was a Monday morning at University of Maryland medical school in Baltimore in the fall of 1948. During a break in classes, a group had gathered. One of the guys was telling about what had happened at a family party the previous Saturday night.

At that time, a Senatorial election was in full swing. The papers were full of pictures of the Democratic candidate shaking hands with a West Coast Communist labor leader. He denied such a meeting had ever occurred.

The Saturday night story being told was that a couple of thugs had come to the party and took away one of his cousins. This young man was brought back later severely beaten. It seems he was the technician in the photographic lab where the picture had been superimposed. He was threatened with his life if he ever told anyone the picture was, indeed, a fake.

For further emphasis, they told him they worked for Senator Joseph McCarthy.

TWO STORIES

In the crush of momentous minutia that
fills the private practice of
Pediatrics, occasionally an episode
makes you pause and reflect. Each time
you happen to think of it, the memory
remains vivid and retains its
emotional impact.

The first of these happened about
sixty years ago. The second has been
with me more than sixty.

(1) Freedom of Information

Among many messages, one day, was one
saying a baby had been born. Normal
pregnancy, labor and delivery. Full-
term. No problems. Another routine
exciting event. The baby was fine. I
visited the mother each day and gave
her instructions about caring for him
when she took him home. She said
nothing to me to indicate she might
have unorthodox ideas about any aspect
of medical practice.

63

The visit at one month showed good growth and development. We discussed some points about feeding and care. She was to return next month. The usual routine, in those days, was to start immunization with DPT and Salk vaccine at that second visit. There seemed no need to discuss this. Thousands of physicians all over the country did the same thing. The child received both shots at that visit.

The third month brought the unexpected.

As I began to examine the child, she said to me: "Did you give my baby a polio shot last month?"

"Why, yes. That's a routine procedure. We've been able to reduce the number of cases of polio drastically with these shots. Now that it's available, we can start this early."

"I don't want you to put any of that junk in my child."

That stopped me.

Many memories shot through my mind. Children wasted and weak, working to breathe. A friend of ours, a lovely girl, who would maneuver the rest of her life on crutches, pulling her metal-brace laden legs and who would painstakingly mount stairs backwards because she had discovered it was easier to do it this way. The very practice I now ran had once been handled by a young pediatrician who, now, could only wiggle a toe as he sat in his wheelchair, totally paralyzed from the neck down and with half the strength of his respiratory muscles gone. Everyone in town had known what had happened to him seven years before. I remembered meeting him through the mirror as he lay in his iron lung -- and remembered part of our first conversation: "It seems amazing, doesn't it," he said, "that if I had taken three little shots, I wouldn't be lying here." Wryly, then: "If I wanted to commit suicide, I couldn't even put a gun to my own head".

65

"Junk! I've given this to my own children, and to hundreds of others as well. This really has changed the whole story of this disease. Besides, you know about the doctor who used to be here. How can you say such a thing?"

"Well, I think it's junk. I read an article in the New York Times that said it causes cancer. So just don't give that to my baby again."

I didn't hide my surprise but nodded assent. Only DPT was injected. She was perfectly pleasant again and we discussed some minor problems. During our last exchange, I requested: "Do you think you could find that Times article? I'd certainly like to see it."

She'd try to find it, and she left. I wondered if I'd ever see her again. The pace of practice caught me up and swept me along.

One month later, she appeared on

schedule.

"There it is."

A New York Times clipping was on my
desk. I noted the headline and read it
carefully. It was a Public Health
Service release intended to reassure
everyone that extreme precautions were
being taken to insure the safety of
every batch of polio vaccine. One of
the ways this was done was to check
every batch for a contaminating virus.
This other virus, the CONTAMINANT,
caused cancer in hamsters. The pure
polio vaccine did NOT. Each lot of
vaccine, therefore, was injected into
test animals. If no cancer occurred,
that lot was approved. If cancer did
occur in the test animals, that lot
was not safe and was discarded.

I finished reading and, trying to
phrase and word as lucidly and gently
as possible, began the interpretation.
Her face became a poker mask.

No response when I finished.

I examined the baby and gave the third
DPT shot -- in silence.

"Have you changed your mind about the
polio shot?"

She dressed the baby and picked him
up. I gave her back the clipping,
which she took, turned, opened the
door and went out without a word. I
knew I would never see her again.

As the door began to close behind her,
a single thought suddenly stunned my
consciousness:

"My God! she has a vote. She is not
stupid but she has seen one or two
words and jumped to a conclusion.
Then, presented with the reality of
more information, she was so angry
with being caught, she refused to
acknowledge anything."

What is the process which closes a
mind after that? It seems to be
selecting only things which support

that conclusion, rejecting or refusing
to examine anything different or that
might differ.

How is a closed mind unlocked?

The key to unlocking is held by each
person themselves. That key is the
question:

"Is that what I do?"

"Is that what I —— "

        (2) THE UNEXPECTED

The other incident comes to mind
whenever anyone discusses "dramatic
impact". Good theater is something my
wife and I have always enjoyed. On a
stage, this incident would probably be
dismissed as "contrived". The
sensation is just as graphic at its
recall today as when I was a first
year Resident in Pediatrics over sixty
years ago.

He was only three years old and we had just confirmed the diagnosis of a brain tumor. His mother was crying hysterically. Several of the doctors had tried to comfort her, but without success. I remember wondering what I would do in the future. Someday, I would be in practice. It was not inconceivable that this could happen to a patient of mine. What would I be able to do for a parent in the same situation? How would I handle such tragic emotion? Such heartache? Reason is a misfit at such a time. Then how?

I didn't see one of the Attending Pediatricians approaching her. My Chief Resident spotted him and nudged me.

"Watch this," he said. He knew what was coming, but I had no idea. This doctor said: "Get a grip on yourself. You don't have to do this. It's not helping you or your child."

It seemed superficial and prosaic.

70

She screamed at him as she had at the others: "How can you tell me such a thing? How do you know what it feels like?"

He spoke quietly and said the one thing she never expected to hear:

"Because I do know what it feels like. My wife and I were able to have only one child and he died of a brain tumor when he was four years old. I'm a Pediatrician and I've spent the rest of my life taking care of other people's children since then --- just as I did before he was born."

As the impact of his words registered, the contortion on her face began to fade. Her jaw dropped slightly as her eyes widened and the sudden silence cut the emotional storm like a knife.

71

"ONLY IF YOU THINK LITERALLY"

In the time before the use of RhoGam, and after the discovery of the Rh antigen (1940) and its relation to erythroblastosis fetalis (1941), an occasional baby was born with a very severe form called "hydrops fetalis". Untreated, there was 100% mortality. Treatment resulted in survival rates between 10% - 30%. In one group of 95 cases of hydrops, 51 were treated but only 8 survived. In reviewing the literature (before computers by using Index Medicus) to report a case I treated with unorthodox methods, I found no reports of the health of the surviving infant and no long-term follow ups on development. When this case was a normally-developed 8 year old girl, a report was indicated. I'm sure many physicians had wondered, as I had, what caused this extraordinary situation. What was different? Why hydrops?

This female infant was born at 1:34 AM on September 20, 1968 after an uneventful pregnancy and weighed 6 lbs 12 oz. She was markedly edematous. After treatment removed the excess fluid, she weighed 4 lbs 7 oz. Thus, at birth, she had half of her true body weight (2 lbs 5 oz) as fluid.

Her mother was O Rh negative. Three previous children were all normal. Back in July, her blood was negative for Rh antibodies. The survival of three normal children was explained by their blood types. The usual situation with Rh incompatibility is that the first child is normal but, subsequent pregnancies, result in either death (unless there is treatment) or retardation. If there is incompatibility but the child is not in much distress at birth, breast feeding transfers more antibodies, which can be absorbed by the newborn stomach, and cause retardation. The Rh antigen has three major components indicated as C D E. D is the main factor. All have lesser alleles indicated as c d e. Though her first child was D (O CDe) the next two were both d: the second was O Cde and the third O cde. This child was A Rh positive CDe. The family was unknown to me prior to the call from the obstetrician at 2: 00 AM.

Her Apgar was 4 based on slow, irregular respirations, heart rate less than 100, color blue and pale with orange-colored amniotic fluid. The enormous and edematous placenta weighed 6 lbs.

There was gross anasarca with pitting edema of head and chest, gross edema of extremities and labia and marked abdominal distention from ascites. Moro weak. Rectal negative. Meconium plug was seen but no meconium passed for three days. Liver was 3 finger breadths below the costal margin and there was splenomegaly.

Cord blood showed a bilirubin of 5.5, Hgb 9.7 with 720 nucleated RBC/100WBC. Polychromatophilia, erythroblasts and proerythroblasts were seen on the smear. Exchange transfusion (500 ml) was begun at 4:45 AM with several episodes of apnea and cyanosis during the exchange, the worst after 400 ml. She responded to nasal suction and manual manipulation of her thoracic cage. After the exchange, she was placed in an Isolette.

By 11:00 AM that morning, edema had increased but jaundice was not obvious, which is common in these cases. Some urine had passed but her chemistries showed blood pH 7.36, pCO2 55 and pO2 40. Flat plate revealed marked ascites and very little intestinal air. I reasoned that the increased intra-abdominal pressure, in addition to preventing ingress of air to the GI tract, could also obstruct renal blood flow, even though a small amount of urine had passed. This could be contributing to the increasing edema. I decided on parascentesis, not knowing, until I'd done a literature search later, that this had been used in hydrops before. My consultants, my Chief of Pediatrics and a surgeon friend, had never done this on an infant less than 24 hours old. The technique that evolved was this: the surgeon suggested an Intracath; as soon as the needle entered the peritoneal cavity, fluid spurted out, -- but the Intracath tube was too small to permit continued drainage. Using my own moiety, I enlarged the opening and introduced a sterile infant gastric feeding tube, turned her onto her right side and taped the tube in place. Then I cut the plug off the other end and placed it through the top of a throat culture tube, taping that to the outside of the Isolette. Fluid poured out so rapidly that a new tube was needed in ten minutes.

By 6:00 PM, her movements had worked the tube out of place but fluid continued to drain from the incision. By 11:00 PM, her abdomen was again becoming distended, though circumference was 1 ½

" less than it had been at birth. Using a groove director as a trochar, another feeding tube was inserted through the incision. As before, fluid spurted out when the peritoneal cavity was entered. Lab data from earlier that afternoon showed bilirubin had gone up to 12.2 and there were now 896 nucleated RBC with Hgb 8.7. Because of her obvious need for increased oxygen-carrying ability, the umbilical vein was re-catheterized so she could get a slow push of 100 cc of O Rh negative packed RBC. I had also prophylactically digitalized her.

Her improvement after that was like a wish-fulfillment fantasy. Next morning, at 32 hours old, her color was good despite persistent marked edema. She was sucking and feeding small amounts on her own, the parascentesis tube was still draining but her Hgb was now 14.7, bilirubin 15.3 and nucleated RBC dramatically dropped to 374.

By the third day, she seemed to be getting tired so she was gavage-fed. Color was still good, urinating freely and abdomen, though large, was now soft. She was 1 lb 8 oz less than her birth weight. The day before, nucleated RBC had been 266 and Hgb 15.8 but by 6:00 AM on this third day, nucleated

RBC were 94 and Hgb16.8, though bilirubin had risen to 17.7. At 2:00 PM, bilirubin was 18.3 but nucleated RBC were only 65.

 On the morning of the fourth day, with bilirubin at 17.7, nucleated RBC were at 22. The first meconium appeared spontaneously --- black, sticky and typical and she was retaining gavage feedings of 30 cc q3h. Palpable edema of the head was gone with edema now only in dependent areas; e.g., labia. By 3:00 PM, nucleated RBC were 8 and she appeared comfortable. Severe hypoproteinemia due to liver damage from the anemia and tissue anoxia is thought to be the cause of the severe edema. The packed RBC transfusion helped to correct that.

7:00 AM on the fifth day saw the Hgb at 15.5 and there were no more nucleated RBC. Bilirubin peaked at 19, was 12.5 the next day and tapered off after that.

Initial throat culture revealed Klebsiella sensitive to ampicillin, which she was given. Throat cultures from myself, the obstetrician and all nursery staff were negative. Since Klebsiella is not always a pathogen, but has been described as a skin contaminant, this was probably the explanation for its presence.

By the next day, edema was much less, respirations normal and she weighed 5.0 lbs. Since the quality and rate of her heart sounds were normal, digitalis was tapered and stopped. Her lowest weight was 4 lbs 7 oz on the ninth day, she was feeding on a nipple and passing normal stools. Discharge was on the 27th day at 5 lbs 1 oz.

Protein electrophoretic studies ruled out the possibility of intrauterine infection. In March 1977 at age 8 ½, she had developed normally including speech and hearing.

The reason for hydrops was still not apparent. One year later, I was curious to know if a double incompatibility (Rh and A-O) might have been the explanation. Repeat antibodies on the mother gave us all a surprise: not only were anti-D levels still high but anti-C levels were even higher. As can be seen from the other children's blood types, this was the second time this mother had had a child with D but the *third* time she'd had one with C. It may be that multiple incompatibilities within the six Rh antigens is the explanation.

In current Pediatric texts, the use of packed RBC in hydrops is a standard recommendation. Back in 1968, figuring through this case was a medical adventure.

POSITION IS EVERYTHING

In recent years, it was found that putting infants on their backs seemed to reduce the incidence of SIDS. Then reports began to appear about the reason we were taught *not* to do this: flattening and distortion of the shape of the head. Actually, lying on the abdomen is a normal and more physiologic position since circulation is easier this way. I remember this being described by the brilliant Dr. William Dock on medical rounds when I was a Rotating Intern at Kings County Hospital in Brooklyn, N.Y. in 1951.

He reminded us all that there is only one place in the heart-lung circulation where the blood is not pumped directly to its intended location: the newly oxygenated blood oozes out of the pulmonary capillaries to the pulmonary veins going to the left atrium. The only pressure is that of the right ventricle pumping venous blood through the pulmonary artery to those capillaries. Since the heart is ventral when the body is prone, gravity helps the flow of blood to the left atrium from the lungs, which are dorsal in this position. When the body is supine, the oxygenated blood must flow upwards against gravity to get to the left atrium.

Then Dr. Dock, with a twinkle in his eyes and a grin, said "-- and Man, in his wisdom, as learned to sleep upon his back".

In the case of an infant, the nose should be suctioned and cleared before being placed on the abdomen and the head carefully turned sufficiently to the side so the nasal passages are unobstructed. These are the "devilish details" which make the difference. This way, the head can be turned alternately to one side or the other preventing pressure distortion anywhere, especially on the occiput.

 If these precautions are observed in positioning the child, I don't think there will be any increase in SIDS, which is an infectious problem. The oldest child I ever saw with SIDS was an 8 year old whose mother called me one morning because she couldn't wake him to get ready for school. He'd been fine the night before. I went to their house immediately, not knowing what I'd find. I had to give her the stunning news but, not wanting to leave her with a dead child, I put him in my car and brought him to the hospital as a DOA. The autopsy confirmed the pulmonary pathology. We presented the case to the famous Dr. Louis Weinstein, who occasionally came down from Boston for consultations at Bridgeport Hospital. His cousin was one of the other pediatricians. He was confounded by this but finally decided, from the pathology findings, that it was SIDS. He said he'd never seen it in anyone this age before. In those days, we put all babies on their abdomen and the large majority did very well. Obviously, position had nothing to do with the problem in the 8 year old.

A NEW CONCEPT OF THE NATURE OF RHEUMATIC
FEVER

In preparation for my year (7/1/1954 –
6/30/1955) as N.Y. State Research Fellow in Rheumatic
Fever at Irvington House, I spent many months reading
bibliography on Rheumatic Fever, streptococcal disease
and antibody responses.   What I am about to present is
a completely different way of attempting to understand
the pathogenesis of this disease.

It is well-established and agreed upon that starting a 10
day course of penicillin within 9 days of the onset of the
strep infection will eradicate the strep and prevent
Rheumatic Fever. From this, I would suggest that
Rheumatic Fever develops after a strep infection when
there is malfunction of the body's *normal* mechanism
for strep eradication.   This is usually accomplished by
the production of anti-M type-specific antibody, the
only strep antibody which gives non-immune white cells
the ability to kill streptococci. Thus, one postulation
might be that the genetic difference which Dr. May

83

Wilson was so convinced must exist in the Rheumatic is the *inability* to produce type-specific anti-M antibody. Is there any basis for such a speculation?

The usual response to the introduction of an antigen, whether by infection or vaccination, is that circulating antigen is usually found for only 9 or 10 days and then antibody appears at about two weeks. Buried in Rothbard's classic article in the J. of Experimental Medicine in 1945 is a passing observation of his surprise at finding circulating M antigen in rheumatic subjects 45 days after the infection. He does not understand this and offers no explanation. Irene Uchida's classical study from Toronto attempting to find some known genetic explanation for the well-documented 2.5% -3.5% incidence of RF after a strep epidemic in the general population was unable to provide an answer.

Is there any evidence for the genetic transfer of the inability to respond to a particular antigen? I found several:

Work done in experimental animals (mice and rabbits) by Sang and Sobey from Scotland (The Genetic Control of Response to Antigenic Stimuli – J. Immunology, 72:1, Jan.1954, p.52) described the genetic transfer of the lack of antibody response in these groups. Stollerman and Siegel followed type-specific antigen (TSA) responses in children after strep infections NOT specifically associated with RF and found TSA responses in 70%. That left 30% with no TSA response. Similarly, Rothbard and Lancefield found 65% of the children in their study developed a TSA response. That means 35% did not.

Behrman, R.E. in "Neonatology Diseases of the Fetus and Infant", 1973, p.185, says "--- a failure of Rh immunization appeared to reflect an inability to respond to the antigen even when it was introduced in substantial quantities. 10% of Rh-negative subjects injected with Rh-positive cells failed to give any antibody response".

The logical next step is visualizing what happens in a person infected with strep which is persistent and not eradicated. The body is now the "culture medium" and production of exotoxin is unopposed. This means larger amounts of streptolysin, hyaluronidase, streptokinase, et al produce larger antibody responses. Many reputable investigators (Rothbard, Watson, Swift, Wilson, Kuttner, Stollerman, Siegel, Harris, Weinstein) have incontrovertibly established that the immune response to strep infection in rheumatic subjects is greater than in those without rheumatic sequellae.

Is there anything in this phenomenon which might explain the destructive changes in connective tissue which are an integral part of the pathology of RF? In Pediatrics 3:482, 1949 there is a paper by Harris, Harris and Nagle (Studies in the Relation of the Hemolytic Streptococcus to Rheumatic Fever ,VI: Comparison of Streptococcal Anti-Hyaluronidase With Antbodies to Other Streptococcal Antigens in the Serum of Patients With RF and Acute Streptococcal Infection: Mucin Clot Prevention Test) in which they not only confirm that

86

strep antibody responses were at least twice as high in rheumatic patients as in non-rheumatics but that anti-hyaluronidase titers were TEN TIMES as high in those with RF. Now picture the body as culture medium flooded by an especially large amount of hyaluronidase in order to achieve that result. Before the antibody response, the action of this enzyme is to digest and destroy hyaluronic acid, the basic component of connective tissue. I would postulate that this is what leads to the fragmentation of collagen fibers and fibrinoid degeneration as the cause of tissue breakdown leading to an inflammatory response.

The development of RF, then, would require the interaction of several variables: an inability to respond to type-specific antigen, a strain producing a large amount of hyaluronidase and, possibly, cross-reactive antigenic similarities. In Dr. James Todd's section on Rheumatic Fever in the 15th Edition of Nelson's Textbook of Pediatrics, he mentions that a group-specific polysaccharide of the Group A strep cell wall is "antigenically similar to the glycoprotein found in

human and bovine cardiac valves". This antibody
against the Group A polysaccharide persists in people
with chronic rheumatic valvular heart disease. I would
wonder if the destruction of the connective tissue of
the valves released this glycoprotein and enhanced the
antibody response to the cell wall polysaccharide. Todd
further states that "When rheumatic mitral valves were
surgically removed and replaced with prosthetic valves,
serum antibody levels against the Group A
polysaccharide fell, as if the antigenic stimulus had been
removed".

 Many things are not clear, however. Antibodies to cell
wall antigens also develop after repeated strep skin
infections, but RF does not appear after pyoderma.

The clinical variants leave much to be answered,
possibly by the molecular geneticists and biologists.
Common antibodies to antigens found in the strep cell
wall and the caudate nucleus of the brain have been
found in Sydenham's chorea. Why are some cases
mainly arthritic or cardiac? Why are these occasionally

found together?   Why the fortunate failure to never find arthritis and chorea in the same patient? Is this related to the difference in the embryological origin from ectodermal and mesodermal layers?

These speculations hardly provide complete answers. Is it possible that strep infection during pregnancy and its bacteremia could allow some M protein to cross the placenta and enter the fetus, thus rendering it immunologically tolerant to that particular M protein? After being born, that child would be unable to eradicate that type of Group A strep infection.

That ought to tickle somebody's imagination!

THREE IDEAS

I.   HOW TO TITER LEUCOCIDIN

In 1954, during my fellowship at
Irvington House, we had a visit from Dr.
Angelo Taranta, who'd been a Fellow
two years before. During lunch, he
described to me a method for making a
slide preparation of living leucocytes.
Put a drop or two of blood on a slide,
put the slide into an open Petri dish
with moistened filter paper on the
bottom and incubate ½ hour. Remove
the slide and wash gently with a pipette
or wash bottle. The red cell clot will
wash off and a film of living leucocytes
will be left on the slide.

During my early years in the practice of Pediatrics, there
was great concern about infection in nurseries with
phage types 80 and 81 coagulase- positive staph aureus.
But how to tell, before the typing, which strain of staph
produced a large amount of leucocidin. That might be

the basis for developing a vaccine. My friend, Dr. Russ Pope, the head of Pathology, gave me a corner of the lab, at Bridgeport Hospital, in which to work during my Wednesday afternoons "off".

A 24 hour broth culture of known coagulase-positive staph aureus (standardized by spectrophotometer) was put through a Seitz filter. A drop of filtrate was put onto the living leucocytes, incubated another half hour and then Wright stained. What I saw was destruction of the leucocyte cell membrane. Some leucocytes were intact, some without the cell membrane and some showed spreading of the granules away from the poly nucleus with the cell membrane gone. This was, obviously, the pathogenetic mechanism: destruction of the body's first line of defense, the polys. Making dilutions of the filtrate to put on the leucocyte preparation made it possible to determine what dilution was required before no membrane destruction was seen.

II. A "NICE" EXPERIMENT TO TEST A THEORY OF "MALIGNANT CHANGE".

In a college genetics course, it was taught that during mitosis, the normal resting electromagnetic charge on the cell membrane was reversed. In a discussion with a Professor of Pathology, I asked whether "malignant change" might be the permanent reversal of this charge thereby creating a condition conducive to constant mitosis with no reversion to the resting state.

He suggested the following: set up a small tank with two electrodes; make suspensions of different kinds of normal cells and different malignant cells. The current generated must be sufficient to get the cells to migrate but not enough to coagulate them once they get to the electrodes. If normal cells and malignant cells migrate to different electrodes, a very fundamental difference would be demonstrated.

I have never had such lab equipment available to me and so have been unable to try this, but have always been curious about what would happen.

III.   RAPID IDENTIFICATION OF THE NATURE OF AN INFECTIOUS PATHOGEN

Though some bacteria can be rapidly identified these days, many still require the 24 hours for culture. In a Yearbook of Pediatrics back in the 1960's, the famous Boston Pediatrician, Dr. Sidney Gellis, described a technique that could quickly give a clinician information about the infecting organism.

Prepare a blood sample for a hematocrit. After spinning down, use filter paper to absorb the supernatant serum. Then carefully pipette the buffy coat and make a gram stain. Since the causative organism will be selectively localized in the leucocytes, it is often possible to at least tell if you're dealing with a gram-positive coccus or a gram-negative rod.

RECURRING PYLORIC STENOSIS

Usually, this resolves after surgery. In practice, I referred to several different excellent surgeons. This particular case went to a father-son team and the baby did well. Two months later, the signs all returned. The parents insisted on going to a University Hospital 20 miles away. They came back having been told that the local surgeons had not done proper surgery.

In discussing this with one of the other surgeons, he explained: "Those two are excellent surgeons. I know what happened because this happened to me. I operated on a baby and it did well. Then symptoms returned. When I did the second surgery, I was amazed. The pylorus looked as though it hadn't been touched but I knew I had cut it properly myself. That's why the academics thought nothing had been done."

As we know, one surgery is usually sufficient. The need for a second does not mean ineptitude.

HARRY GREEN'S LOST WORK

In the fall of 1949, our Junior Class heard a lecture by Dr. Harry Green, a pathologist at Yale, describing his most fascinating and original work.

In the 1930s, it was customary to use carcinogenic agents on lab animals and then try to treat these. But these were rat or rabbit cancers. Dr. Green wanted to find a way to grow human cancers in lab animals so any effective therapy would be valid for humans.

Somehow, he discovered that the anterior chamber of the eye was a natural tissue-culture medium nourished by the living animal. This led to the amazing discovery that, after a week growing in the eye, the biopsy of malignant tissue lost its tissue specificity and could be transplanted to the leg or abdomen of the animal without being rejected. It could even be transplanted to a different animal or, even, a different species: e.g., grown in the eye of a guinea pig a carcinoma could be transplanted to the leg of a rabbit. In addition, anaplastic malignancies would often grow and reveal their tissue of origin. (They did not have today's molecular techniques.) The only inconsistent finding was that biopsies of leukemic nodes would not take and grow. For me, this correlated with something I'd noted as students when we were studying hematology: they'd look for a leukemic patient to show us the immature stages in leucocyte evolution, the normal immature stages. I wondered if leukemia were a disease of interrupted maturation. A proper number of normal leucocytes would signal the bone marrow to slow production. Without such a signal, the marrow would be continually putting out proleucocytes, never getting a signal that there were enough mature ones.

He also found that normally differentiated and benign tumor tissue would not take and grow in the eye.

Knowing the similarity between malignant and embryonic tissue, he asked the surgeons doing abortions to give him the embryos. Not only would embryonic tissue grow in the eye, but if anlage of a system were put there, he could watch the normal maturation exactly as it would have proceeded in utero.

He saw kidney anlage grow into kidney with a ureter. Curiosity led him to do a PSP test and he found, indeed, the kidney was functioning. (If this were possible today, it could allow renal transplants without the need for constant anti-rejection medication, as growth in the eye medium would cause the loss of tissue specificity.)

Growing lung gave him another surprise. The prevailing theory, at that time, was that the lung expanded with the child's first breath. He couldn't understand why, when sectioned, the lung — which obviously hadn't been exposed to air — had distended alveoli. No one knew about surfactant then.

He also found an inexpensive pregnancy test. When ovarian anlage matured to an ovary, he could watch a follicle ovulate if a drop of pregnant urine were put into the animal's conjunctival sac. Not pregnant. No ovulation. With a normal ovary having hundreds of eggs, the potential is obvious. He said he'd brought this to several pharmaceutical companies but no one was interested.

I heard him three years later when I was a first-year Pediatric Resident at Maimonides Hospital in Brooklyn, N.Y. At that time, he had three patients: one diabetic and two Addison's. All had transplants of the needed tissue in their abdominal muscles. The Addison's were doing fine. The diabetic had done without any therapy for 4 months and then the pancreatic tissue had begun to deteriorate. He was investigating why this had happened but had no explanation at that time. This was 1953. I watched the literature for the publication of his work and to see if he'd found an explanation for the pancreatic tissue failure.

A few years later, I heard that he'd died. I couldn't understand why such creative research never got published. Much later in life, by pure chance, I stumbled on the answer.

After 18 years in the private practice of Pediatrics, I spent 9 years in ER and then received an offer in Occupational Medicine. I started at Union Carbide's Medical Department at their World Headquarters in Danbury, CT. The explosion at the Carbide plant in Bhopal, India, led to the break-up of that huge corporation. That's when I became Medical Director of Chesebrough-Pond's/Unilever, USA. In this position, I was responsible for product testing to assure product safety. One of my responsibilities was to attend the Johns Hopkins two-day seminar in Baltimore on Alternative Methods of Product Testing (i.e., without using animals).

It was there I heard a presentation by Dr. Eugene Bell, a Ph.D. from MIT, who ran a testing lab which used artificially-grown human skin. They started with newborn circumcised foreskins and were also trying to grow a circulatory system. Wanting to investigate this further, my Manager of Product Safety (a 30 year Chesebrough chemist) and I arranged a visit to the lab which, at that time, was in Cambridge, MA.

When Bell and his associates finished their presentations, it so much reminded me of Dr. Green's work, I began telling him about it. I finished by expressing my disappointment at not having seen the work published. My last words were "I wonder whatever happened to Harry Green's notes?". With a big grin, Bell said "I've got Harry Green's notes. I knew him well." I realized he'd used those notes to start this lab and never allowed Green to get the credit for all his brilliant and imaginative work. In my official position and in his lab, I could not say what I thought of him but vowed I would write the story of this egregious research injustice. I regret it has taken me so long to do so.

www.ingramcontent.com/pod-product-compliance
Lightning Source LLC
Chambersburg PA
CBHW070327190526
45169CB00005B/1772